*Can Vitamin E prevent
heart disease?*

Can Vitamin E heal burns?

Can I take iron with Vitamin E?

*What is my daily requirement
of Vitamin E?*

These questions and their authoritative answers are among the many in this comprehensive survey of Vitamin E, prepared by Dr. Evan V. Shute, renowned for his pioneering use of the vitamin in successful treatment of a wide range of conditions.

This new, enlarged edition of this popular book presents 50 new questions and answers, covering everything you need to know about the substance that has saved, enriched, and prolonged many lives—and may do the same for yours.

Common Questions on Vitamin E and Their Answers

Evan V. Shute, F.R.C.S. (C)

Keats Publishing, Inc. New Canaan, Connecticut

COMMON QUESTIONS ON VITAMIN E
AND THEIR ANSWERS

Pivot Health Book edition published 1979

ISBN: 0-87983-191-X
Library of Congress Catalog Card Number: 79-87677

Printed in the United States of America

PIVOT BOOKS are published by Keats Publishing, Inc.
36 Grove Street, New Canaan, Connecticut 06840

Foreword

We have compiled over 100 of the most commonly encountered questions concerning vitamin E, and the doctors of the Shute Institute, at London, Canada, have drafted short answers to them. These we are hereby publishing in book form, for ready reference and in order to help you give authoritative answers quickly and with a minimum of clerical work.

Throughout this book the authors have used the term vitamin E at one time and the proper scientific term, alpha tocopherol, at another time. The agent that is being described is the same in each case. "Vitamin E" is a sort of medical slang for a set of seven tocopherols, one of them, called alpha tocopherol, being the active agent for cardio-vascular patients. For all practical purposes vitamin E is a term interchangeable with alpha tocopherol, and is often used in place of the latter because it is so much better known.

We hope you will find this little book helpful. It should be read in conjunction with an earlier book, *The Heart and Vitamin E*, also published by the Shute Foundation and Keats Publishing.

Table of Contents

Tocopherol (To Cope for All)
An Appreciation of Dr. Evan V. Shute ix

Introduction xi

What Is Vitamin E? xv

An Ounce of Prevention xx

Heart 1

Circulatory Diseases of the Legs 41

Uses in Obstetrics, Gynecology, Urology
and Pediatrics 59

Diabetes Mellitus 67

Miscellaneous Uses 71

General Aspects of Vitamin E 83

-------------------------------*Tocopherol*

To Cope For All!   Dr. Evan Shute

It was the enthusiastic dedication of this man to collect, correlate and collate all to be known and all to be learned about Vitamin E. His research was International, and his life was an encyclopedia of the fruits of his efforts.

The legacy of his work has been and will continue to be a foundation for others to build upon.

This anti-oxidant, protector from peroxidation, defier of rancidity, free radical scavenger, lipid stabilizer . . . its one guiding biochemical property . . . so applicable to so many areas of man's biological being and clinical needs. He laid the cornerstone.

Robert E. Fishbein, M.D.
New York City, 1979

No substance known to medicine has such a variety of healing properties as alpha tocopherol (vitamin E). It is unique. That has always been one of its major difficulties: It is too useful for too many things.

One would never expect, in the day of the antibiotics or tranquilizers or cortisone, that the possession of multiple values would be a hindrance to the acceptance of alpha tocopherol, but it is.

Medical men who were originally taught that alpha tocopherol was a "fertility vitamin," controlling the tendency to miscarry noticed in some women, later learned to their surprise that it could resolve scars in claw-like hands, and often refused to believe it was more useful still for diseases of the heart and blood vessels. That was too much.

All important medical discoveries have sounded improbable or even a bit fantastic to both doctors and laymen alike. Think back on some of the older discoveries and how odd they must have seemed at first. Fancy taking a mold from the air, growing it on artificial media, then injecting a solution containing it into muscle to treat an overwhelming bacterial infection in the abdomen, lungs or tonsils! It sounded so fantastic that it took fourteen years and the Second World War for medical men to *give it a trial*! However, we have all conveniently forgotten our first misgivings in our current enthusiasm for penicillin.

Insulin is but one of a host of similar examples. Imagine extracting a fluid from the pancreas of a slaughtered animal and injecting it under the skin of humans to help the body use any sugar not properly handled by the patient's own pancreas. That is what Sir Frederick Banting did and then announced the fluid to the medical world as insulin.

Alpha tocopherol (vitamin E) was at first received with the same unbelief and for the same reasons. Once understood, however, it will be as universally used as are the antibiotics (penicillin or streptomycin, tetracycline) and insulin.

Vitamin E is useful for a variety of diseases which at first seem totally unrelated. But there is one factor that they have in common—a local decrease in oxygen supply because of injury to veins, arteries or capillaries, or because of internal organ derangements. Understand this, and the reasons become obvious for the use of tocopherol in such apparently dissimilar conditions as nephritis, coronary thrombosis, burns and diabetes mellitus.

Skepticism is no new thing. The difficulties encountered by penicillin we have already cited. One would have thought its virtues were obvious from the first, and readily demonstrable. BCG vaccine, after clinical trials made upon millions of people over the last fifty years, still has an uncertain future. The use of anticoagulants in coronary heart disease, even after a carefully controlled study carried out by hundreds of the leading medical men of 16 university hospitals on 1031 patients has been followed by scores more.

One can go back further into medical history and recall the story of X ray. When X rays were discovered morality brigades were formed at once, designed to resist such a destruction of decency and privacy. A London firm made a small fortune selling X-ray-proof underwear. An attempt was made in New York to legislate against the use of X rays in opera glasses in theatres. All this is now forgotten, but it illustrates that some of the best medical advances have had tardy recognition.

Such medical and public caution is wise, particularly in a day like ours when medical advances are so numerous and, like the Salk vaccine for polio, often take long to adjudicate. But once the evidence accumulates to the height that studies on alpha tocopherol have reached, and when the diseases it can alleviate and prevent are so menacing and general, the debate should not be prolonged further. For in the meantime thousands upon thousands suffer or die needlessly while easy help lies within their reach.

Hence this little book. We want to be sure that the medical profession, as well as the patients dependent on it, know what help is available. We have spent many years in bringing our findings before doctors. We have published a profusely illustrated textbook on the subject for scientists and medical men in general. We have lectured on our findings before the British, Canadian and Ontario Medical Associations and the National Medical Association of the United States, as well as before many international medical meetings. This is the customary procedure with new medical observations, and this custom we have observed. Now here are the facts in everyday language.

Vitamins have always been labeled according to the letters of the alphabet. This was a good device as long as it was a simple matter of A,B,C and D. Now since there are M,P, and even lower letters in the series, and, what is worse, several D vitamins and even more B vitamins, this system of nomenclature has aroused much criticism. Whenever possible, scientists now differentiate the components of the vitamin B complex by speaking of thiamine chloride or riboflavin or pantothenic acid or niacin. They even prefer to speak of ascorbic acid in place of vitamin C, although only one type of C is known.

Vitamin E is also a complex of several factors: the alpha, beta, gamma, delta, epsilon, eta and zeta tocopherols. For all practical purposes gamma and delta, perhaps epsilon, can be ignored at the moment. Alpha, beta and zeta appear to be the factors of most use to us in medicine, and alpha overshadows the rest. Hence in this book we equate vitamin E to alpha tocopherol, since "vitamin E" is merely a kind of medical shorthand or slang for the alpha substance.

What is a vitamin? It is a food factor, present

in minute amounts in certain foods we eat, and essential for proper nutrition. Each one of the many so far discovered acts in a way characteristic for it and for no other. It may act on one set of tissues only, perhaps on one small focus in the body. Some, it is true, have certain resemblances to one another in their effects, for example, alpha tocopherol and pyridoxine (a fraction of vitamin B). Some are helpful to one another or, as we say, "synergistic." An example of good companions are vitamin A and alpha tocopherol. Some are antagonistic, such as alpha tocopherol and natural vitamin D (because of the unsaturated fats in fish liver oils, the commonest source of D).

For a long time vitamins were supposed to be harmless in any amount. Now it is known that overdoses of such factors as nicotinic acid (part of the B fraction) or vitamin D can be given to certain susceptible persons, and that a high dosage of ascorbic acid (vitamin C) may be poorly tolerated by some stomachs. High doses of the tocopherols may develop the same problem, or produce diarrhea or a skin rash. Some people have trouble taking thiamine.

Presumably most vitamins take part in the activity of the enzyme systems of the body. Recent work, for example, suggests that alpha tocopherol is involved in the activities of such a substance, called cytochrome C. In the heart it is involved in enzyme systems of a complex nature called nucleotidases and oxidases. As yet these biochemical processes are far from adequately explored. Suffice it to say that vitamins appear to be potent in small quantities, are essential to the enzyme systems of the body, and are often involved in an integral way in the metabolism of foods.

Vitamin E (alpha tocopherol) is known to act as an anti-oxidant, hindering the undue or too-rapid oxidation of fats. It hinders the production of tissue peroxides, hence the deposition in tissue of pigment "clinkers" (incompletely burned or oxidized food factors). It is also a factor in the utilization of both carbohydrates and proteins, the other main constituents of all food.

In recent years the concept has evolved of the use of vitamins as drugs, without regard to their activities in minute quantities in food. Thus *huge* doses of vitamin D, far beyond those ordinarily demanded by the body, have been used by physicians treating arthritis. Huge doses of vitamin C have been used in an anti-infective role. Huge doses of niacin have been used as a dilator of blood vessels. Huge doses of thiamine chloride and of B-1 have been used for neuritis. This involves the so-called "pharmacodynamic" action of these substances—in short their use as drugs, not as replacement only. It is in this sense that we usually administer vitamin E nowadays, especially for cardiovascular conditions, using doses far larger than the so-called "minimum daily requirement." This has opened up a whole new field in vitamin therapy, which is no longer regarded as being of value purely for the relief of major deficiencies or for replacement. We are now in the epoch of *"megavitamins"* (as christened by Professor Linus Pauling).

Since the exact chemical structure of many vitamins is now known, some have been made synthetically to set beside those isolated from natural sources. Most of our early clinical work was done with synthetic alpha tocopherol, for example. We learned from this experience that it was the alpha fraction of vitamin E that was most significant therapeutically. Probably synthetic ascorbic acid is now more widely used than natural vitamin C. Certainly synthetic vitamin K is used almost exclusively, since new K-like substances have been found to be more potent than the natural vitamin K originally discovered. Not only that, but knowledge of the structure formulae of vitamins has enabled researchers to predict that substances with somewhat similar molecular configurations might duplicate some or all of the roles that certain vitamins play. Hence the interesting studies indicating how far selenium, methylene blue or diphenyl-p-phenyl-enediamine can replace alpha tocopherol, for instance.

Vitamins can act much like hormones, alpha tocopherol resembling progesterone in its effect on pregnancy, for example. Or they can be antagonistic, just as a female sex hormone and vitamin E have very different effects upon the vaginal wall or blood clots in the legs. Unravelling the chemical nature of these agents has gone far to indicate the parts they play, occasionally has enabled man to improve them, and certainly has suggested more and more roles in which they may prove valuable.

We have always been more interested in prevention than in cure. Why should men wait to be stricken with degenerative diseases when there is now good hope of warding off many of them or of ameliorating the bad effects of such as are already well under way?

Admittedly, one cannot ward off broken legs but must take them as they come. One cannot ward off pneumonia, perhaps, or the lightning bolt. But medicine has gradually developed immunizations against many such infectious diseases as smallpox and diptheria, and lately antibiotics have come to our aid to combat infection in general as soon as it shows its ugly face. The degenerative diseases remain largely untouched—and we age, develop hardened arteries and brains, lose our hair and our sight, notice our skin wrinkle and sag as if Medicine had nothing to say about all this.

We believe that there is now hope for the cardiovascular degenerations, at least. We all know what alpha tocopherol can do for these conditions once they have developed. And the outstanding characteristic of such food factors as the vitamins is that they prevent what they relieve. In short, why wait for your coronary? Why not prevent it?

One uses vitamin B-1 to prevent neuritis because it has been found to cure neuritis.

One uses vitamin B-2 to prevent catilosis, which has such symptoms as raw tongue and lips and indicates B-2 (riboflavin) deficiency.

One uses niacin to prevent pellagra because it has been found so valuable in treating pellagra.

One uses vitamin C to prevent scurvy because it has long been known to cure scurvy.

One uses vitamin D to prevent rickets because it has long been known to cure rickets.

One uses vitamin K to prevent hemorrhagic disease of the newborn because it cures hemorrhagic disease of the newborn.

Could vitamin E (alpha tocopherol) be the sole exception to the rule that vitamins tend to prevent what they relieve?

Here is the most helpful thing to be said about the prevention of these cardiovascular degenerative diseases since they were first recognized.

We know statistically that coronary heart disease kills an increasing number each year. Does one take a bigger chance awaiting his coronary clot or taking out the insurance policy that is alpha tocopherol?

People complain: "Does everyone need to take alpha tocopherol? Isn't this treatment too expensive? If I take it, will I ever be able to discontinue its use?"

We think that everyone needs alpha tocopherol. In some instances it is vitally important, such as for the maintenance routine of any diabetic. Alpha tocopherol costs no more than other food, and life is cheap at the price. Of course, one must take it as long as he lives, just as one would continue eating any other food item. We know no other factor more versatile nor more valuable in the body's economy.

Common Questions on Vitamin E and Their Answers

Heart

Q. 1 — *What are the symptoms of angina pectoris?*

A.—Angina pectoris means pain in the chest, but the term is usually restricted to indicate pain in the heart. It is pain inside the chest, *not in the chest wall*. Therefore, it is *not* brought on by coughing, by turning in bed, by taking a deep breath, and is *not* associated with tender spots on the chest wall. Such symptoms as these mean that the chest muscles or nerves are at fault, or there is pleurisy, but do *not* refer to the heart.

Heart pain occurs when the heart is put to work by exertion or excitement, and occurs only on such exertion, disappears at rest, and recurs when the exertion or excitement recurs. It develops in a heart crying out in pain when deprived of enough oxygen for its activities. It is usually believed to indicate thickening of the coronary arteries which supply the heart muscle. They do so inadequately if they are slowly made smaller by the thickening of the arterial walls.

There is a nocturnal angina, too, but this is rarer.

Chest pain can occur coincidentally with true angina, but the two should be differentiated, and usually it is easy to do so, as suggested above.

Q. 2 — *What is demanded in the treatment of angina pectoris?*

A.—Either more circulation or more oxygen is needed by the starved heart muscle, or there should be less activity on the part of the patient. This last can be achieved both by rest and by avoiding excitement. When smaller demands are made on a damaged heart it may still be able to meet them without producing anginal pain.

But few people can or will lessen their activities voluntarily. Men must work and women must sweep. It is hard to earn money at rest, and the rent must still be paid.

Therefore as an alternative we try to stimulate circulation in the coronary vessels. The patient can get relief from nitroglycerine or peritrate or other such substances, which temporarily dilate the coronary blood vessels. This does nothing, however, for long-range treatment, or for the underlying cause of the circulatory blockade.

Vitamin E (alpha tocopherol) does much more for such a heart by getting at the basic difficulty, as is explained below.

Q. 3 — *What are the symptoms of a coronary attack?*

A.—There may be no symptoms; many a coronary attack is recognized only by an electrocardiogram taken for other reasons, or at postmortem examination.

However, the usual picture is one of severe and sudden heart or chest pain, accompanied by varying degrees of heart failure and shock, often by death. There can be transient fever and elevated white count, prostration, "acute indigestion," pallor, sweating and other evidences of "shock"—but the outstanding symptom is severe heart pain, which may remain for days, or come and go, and be totally or nearly totally incapacitating.

The physician can recognize the *probable* diagnosis, and within a few days can confirm or disprove it by means of an electrocardiogram.

Q. 4 — *To what extent can vitamin E restore health after a heart attack or stroke?*

A.—Under skilled supervision where all the variables are under control, and assuming compliance on the part of the patient, vitamin E is life insurance to these cases. The extent of restoration is primarily dependent on time. It takes thirty years for some chronic deficiencies to manifest themselves in physical disease; it must be realized that it can take as long to correct a deficiency as it does to make it.

Q. 5 — *What are the symptoms of hypertensive heart disease?*

A.—Hypertension (elevated blood pressure) of long standing, plus evidence of gradual and increasing heart failure. By heart failure one means increasing shortness of breath, swelling of the ankles and legs, swelling of the liver, fluid in the lungs, and increasing weakness and inability to move about or to do work.

Q. 6 — *If a patient has hypertensive heart disease, what can he do to help himself?*

A.—Consult a physician at once, in the hope that he can lower the blood pressure safely and wisely and reduce the evidences of heart failure by means of diuretics, digitalis and alpha tocopherol. He should live within his decreased limits, and avoid worry, anger and excitement since these tend to elevate his blood pressure. He should regain a more normal weight if obese. It may be that a diet low in animal fats will be suggested or one to which corn oil is added, in the hope of minimizing further hardening of his arteries. Since our knowledge of diet is in such flux at the moment, perhaps no real alteration of diet will be advised until more is known. Remember that by this time any hardening of the arteries that contributed to the symptoms has already got well underway, and it is dubious if any restriction of further sclerotic processes that one could achieve by dietary or other measures would alter the situation appreciably. Why torture the patient needlessly, therefore, by dietary restrictions which are of uncertain value and where medical recommendations are at present based upon a great deal of conflicting data?

7

Q. 7 — *What are the symptoms of rheumatic heart disease?*

A.—Rheumatic heart disease may start with acute rheumatic fever or imperceptibly. Many cases, therefore, are never recognized until many years afterward.

Acute rheumatic fever is very characteristic; a fever with acutely tender, swollen, painful joints. The joint pain "wanders" from one joint to another, the *wandering* being characteristic of this disease. A heart murmur may develop and there may be listlessness and illness out of all proportion to the fever and its obvious features. Gradually, with or without treatment, the attack subsides.

The patient may remain comparatively well for years thereafter, only in later life developing evidence of heart damage, such as murmurs, with increasing evidences of failure due to softened or scarred heart muscle. This chronic, increasing heart failure, in the absence of high blood pressure or coronary disease, suggests that a chronic rheumatic process has been under way for many years. Deterioration is usually steady thereafter, despite such drugs as diuretics or digitalis, unless vitamin E can stay its course.

Q. 8 — If a patient has rheumatic heart disease, what should he do about it?

A.—If he has acute rheumatic fever, salicylates (aspirin and its relatives) relieve the joint pains and may do some good to the heart itself. Cortisone derivatives are now regarded as questionable in respect to their long-range results; however, they tend to suppress the acute symptoms temporarily. Rest in bed is advised because that decreases the stress put on a damaged heart. We always advise vitamin E because it is a muscle tonic needed by that tired heart muscle, minimizes scar (which matters to a heart that tends to develop valve scarring), may shrink spots of scarring already developed in the heart muscle, and oxygenates the tissues, whose circulation is beginning to flag; nothing else can help here.

Chronic rheumatic heart disease is discussed on pages 11, 24, 27, 28, 29, 39, 65, 92.

Q. 9 — Can anything be done for a congenital heart?

A.—A great deal is now done for such hearts. Indeed, heart surgery has become one of the most active fields in all surgery, regularly shows a great deal of progress, and deals very largely with just such defects.

However, operations for all types of congenital heart disease have not yet been devised and many patients may always lie outside the realm of surgery.

For these, indeed for all congenital hearts, vitamin E offers unique help. It improves tissue oxygenation and hence the patient's color and breathlessness. It improves muscle tone and hence the crippled heart's efficiency. It is of great benefit in preparing these patients for operation, as experience has shown, and in their post-operative convalescence, particularly in patients where operation has proved less satisfactory than was hoped.

Q. 10 — *What can one do to prevent heart disease?*

A.—*Congenital heart disease may* be prevented by giving alpha tocopherol to the sire before conception. There is now good evidence that if the husband's sperms are invigorated by the use of alpha tocopherol before conception occurs, the subsequent child is much more apt to be perfectly formed.

Rheumatic heart disease is largely a response to infection by a particular strain of the streptococcus. This organism is very common and is apt to infect the patient after tonsillitis and other upper respiratory infections. Control of this strain of streptococcus by the steady use of penicillin or sulpha drugs should do much to prevent rheumatic infection. However, the patient's resistance is just as important as the infectious assault, and this we know little about. "Good health," whatever that is, may be as important in prevention as any other factor.

Once infection has occurred, penicillin or sulpha is very helpful, if properly and continually administered. But vitamin E also has much to offer, as suggested above, both in preventing scarring in the heart muscle and the heart valves, in strengthening flabby heart muscle, and in providing better oxygenation of tissues and restoring the integrity of the walls of damaged capillaries. It should be taken for years after the acute attack, because the rheumatic process is insidious and often shows itself five to ten years after the initial bout of rheumatic fever.

Hypertensive and Arteriosclerotic Heart Disease appear to be degenerative processes, usually associated with high blood pressure. Controlling weight, nervous tension and hypertension is helpful, undoubtedly, although it is easier to make these suggestions than to carry them out. Some families have more of a tendency to this disease than others, and members of such families should be especially careful. This is also true of people with diabetes, underactive thyroids, and the rarer conditions usually associated with high values of blood cholesterol.

Much has been written on the pros and cons of cholesterol in these heart diseases and especially coronary heart disease, but medical men are still very unsure of their ground here. Perhaps there is more to be gained by avoiding obesity and undue mental stress, reducing animal fats in the diet and maintaining physical activity than by paying attention to cholesterol. We never do blood cholesterol estimations unless asked to do so, and pay little or no attention to the cholesterol theories of atherosclerosis, believing instead in the rival theory of Professor Duguid. He contends that thickening of the arteries is due to the repeated deposition of small clots on the vessel linings, these clots gradually building up and becoming incorporated into the vessel walls to thicken them. If his theories are substantiated— and the evidence is strong—then cholesterol is merely a secondary invader and not a primary causative factor at all.

Coronary Heart Disease prevention is one of the major medical problems of our time. Here is a disease that has been recognized for nearly 190 years, that has been characterized by sudden clots causing death for about sixty years (these have been recognized clinically only since 1912), and which now is the commonest killer stalking our continent. More work has been done on its prevention and cure than on any comparable disease but cancer or polio or tuberculosis, and still it runs rampant through civilized lands. Probably it is of dietary origin, but the evidence for this is indirect and vague. Its rise corresponds with a method of milling wheat which rejects most or all of the germ, but also with the rise of the cigarette habit and the increase of motor exhaust gases. Perhaps all of these play a causative role. The mental stress of our day has also been blamed, but I believe this underestimates the stress under which our pioneer forefathers lived who were not coronary victims. It still remains true that we are better able to treat it than to prevent it. Unfortunately, many cases of coronary occlusion never survive the first attack, which is why prevention is so much more desirable than mere treatment.

Our experience stresses the value of alpha tocopherol here, too, for it may prevent blood from coagulating inside the vessels, and may also be Nature's own anticoagulant in the circulation. It provides and maintains collateral circulation about vessels that are becoming blocked by the "hardening" process. It maintains the integrity of vessel walls. It dissolves clots already formed, and may, indeed, prevent or resolve microscopic "sludging" in the capillaries. It improves tissue oxygenation and hence local tissue resistance. We now have evidence that it increases the longevity of those who have already had coronary occlusions, and hence should always be considered in the prophylaxis of such recurrent attacks.

In general, one should advise patients who want to avoid heart attacks to be active and not sluggish, to maintain normal weight and avoid becoming fat, to take alpha tocopherol daily in large doses, even from babyhood, and to learn to live with the stresses of our day—to develop a calm philosophy, in other words.

Q. 11 — *What is "arteriosclerosis"?*

A.—That term refers to hardened arteries. The walls thicken, lose their elasticity, can become calcified to resemble goose quills or tiny pipes, and develop tiny lumps or streaks on their linings which often contain cholesterol and other lipids. The process can be patchy throughout the body, and may be largely restricted to the aorta, the great vessel leading all the blood out of the left side of the heart, or may concentrate on the vessels of the brain, of the eyes, or in the coronaries, or in the vessels of the thigh, calf or foot. Generally, however, the process attacks in a number of places at once, some being more advanced than others for reasons not completely clear to us. It is generally a disease of the elderly, although many old people seem to escape it, and more and more young men display it.

Q. 12 — *Does vitamin E have anything to offer for arteriosclerosis?*

A.—Yes, a great deal.

Arteriosclerosis is not a disease confined to man, although it appears to be largely a disease of civilization and harasses men more than women. It is particularly liable to develop in diabetics and patients with decreased activity of the thyroid gland, and in certain families predisposed to high blood values of cholesterol.

But it has recently been found to affect other animals, notably hens. The disease in hens is not unlike that in man. In these creatures a combination of vitamins A and E has proved very effective in both preventing and in relieving the manifestations of arteriosclerosis. Possibly this applies to man as well, and we act on that assumption.

Whatever the direct or indirect effect of alpha tocopherol on the atherosclerotic process in human blood vessels, certainly vitamin E has much to offer patients who have already developed symptoms of arteriosclerosis, such as leg cramps on exertion (claudication), or cold feet, or gangrene, or angina pectoris. Unfortunately, it has very little if anything to offer for hardening of the arteries in the brain (cerebral arteriosclerosis), perhaps because this cannot be recognized before irreparable destruction of brain tissue has developed, and brain tissue is unable to regenerate once it has been damaged.

We doubt if it acts directly on the great arteriosclerotic vessels when it is used in treating the lesions that arise from hardened arteries.

Perhaps it merely mobilizes some of the vast reserves of unused blood vessels we all have and thus enables blood by means of circulatory detours to by-pass the roadblocks in the circulation produced by the arteriosclerotic process as it limes up the great arteries. Such a process has been demonstrated when the principal arteries to the limbs or heart have been tied off in experimental animals, and is almost certainly the mechanism of relief in arteriosclerotic obstructions in man. We all have more brain, more heart, more liver, more kidney, and more lung than we need for survival. Hence one can cut out a lung or kidney and the patient goes on as before. In the same way we have great reserves of unused blood vessels to be called on in emergency or as we grow older. These are mobilized by alpha tocopherol as by nothing else we know, and so can preserve tissues otherwise deprived of adequate arterial circulation.

Tissues cheated of circulation are automatically tissues deprived of oxygen and therefore apt to give pain (as in angina of the heart or claudication in the leg). Pain can be relieved there only by supplying those parts with oxygen. Vitamin E is uniquely able to do this, for it has special powers of enabling the body tissues to make better use of what oxygen they receive. This is really equivalent to providing them with more oxygen. In short, alpha tocopherol helps tissues to breathe, and this can be vital in relieving tissue pain or improving functional activity. In fact, it may make the difference between the life and death of a tissue or even of a person.

Q. 13 — *Would arteriosclerosis be prevented if one took alpha tocopherol regularly from child-hood on?*

A.—No one knows.

No one knows what causes arteriosclerosis, indeed, although various rival theories are to the fore. It is very hard, therefore, to postulate a means of prevention when one does not know the mechanism one is trying to help or hinder.

All one can accurately say is that arteriosclerotic *complications* are greatly and uniquely helped by the use of alpha tocopherol, and that food factors regularly prevent pathological conditions they relieve. Thus one prevents rickets by giving cod liver oil because cod liver (vitamin D) cures rickets. Similarly vitamin C prevents the scurvy it relieves, and vitamin B_1 does the same for neuritis, and vitamin A for xerophthalmia and vitamin K for hemorrhagic disease of the newborn. Would vitamin E be the only exception to this general rule for food factors, even for such agents as calcium or iron?

We believe that every person should always take alpha tocopherol (vitamin E).

Q. 14 — *Is lack of circulation in the thigh causing cramps running down to the metatarsal arch due to a form of arteriosclerosis? If so, will vitamin E help?*

A.—Arteriosclerotic legs tend to cramp on walking. The cramps disappear with rest. This is not to be confused with the agonizing cramp in the leg in bed which pulls up the toes or produces tender knots and leaves the leg tender the next day. This last is ascribable to calcium deficiency and is not circulatory in origin.

Vitamin E improves circulation in legs where the arteries are closing up with arteriosclerosis. It does this by providing detour channels around the blocked or plugged arteries, thus enabling semi-starved tissues to do better on what nutriment they do receive.

Q. 15 — *Is a low cholesterol diet advisable with vitamin E?*

A.—As we have said, we are more impressed by the studies of Duguid's school in England than we are with the American high cholesterol theory of the origin of vascular sclerosis. On that account we pay very little attention to cholesterol in our patients' diets. It is known, for instance, that if cholesterol is restricted in the diet the body still produces a good deal of cholesterol on its own. If one plans to restrict cholesterol he actually should insist on a cholesterol-*free* diet rather than a *low* cholesterol diet. It is very questionable if the low cholesterol diet is as efficient as it might seem at first sight, and that one can continue it indefinitely, decade after decade.

There is a tremendous amount of investigation in process in this particular field at the moment and we soon should know much more definitely than we do now what is the real relationship between cholesterol in the diet and hardening of the arteries.

Q. 16 — *How long does it take vitamin E to give relief in angina?*

A.—Usually it takes several weeks before patients

feel much relief from their angina after they begin taking alpha tocopherol. There are many patients who require much longer than that. This probably depends upon the degree of arterial sclerosis, the degree of deprivation of blood and consequent anemia in the local heart wall, but most of all upon the presence or absence of an extensive collateral (detour) circulation. If thickening of the coronary artery develops gradually over the course of years the circulatory system may compensate for the gradual deficiency of local circulation by opening up a network of small communicating channels between the involved branch and adjacent intact branches of the coronary artery; the result is that any anemic area of painful heart muscle is supplied by secondary channels rather than by the diminishing primary channel, and becomes less anemic and less painful, if painful at all. If the sclerotic process gives time for this compensation to become quite efficient the circulation may remain adequate for years. However, if the circulatory obstruction has come on quickly, and no arterial detours have already had time to form, then alpha tocopherol stimulates new pathways to form as no other drug can, and helps to maintain circulatory equilibrium even in the face of a grave assault upon it.

On the other hand, there is always the question of how much the patient expects to do. It is easier to relieve angina in a man who is not testing his heart too severely than it is to relieve angina in a man who is lifting sacks of flour or climbing mountains or walking on catwalks.

Q. 17 — *Is it advisable for a person with past experience of a slight anginal pain to use vitamin E as a preventative of future trouble?*

A.—Certainly anybody who has ever had angina pectoris should use vitamin E. It is almost equivalent to putting an aqualung on that man's back because it enables his tissues to utilize oxygen better, and those heart tissues vitally need oxygen. That is why they cry out in pain when they are being cheated of it on account of hardened coronary arteries. Vitamin E also helps to produce collateral circulation. This has been very clearly shown in experiments done in Spain, where investigators tied off the coronary artery in dogs and then saw an effective collateral circulation develop around the site of the obstruction when alpha tocopherol was given to the animals. This is Nature's effort to re-supply blood to an area which has been temporarily deprived of it.

Then, too, vitamin E tends to prevent clotting in the blood vessels. People with anginal pain usually fear coronary thrombosis. Here is the cheapest and simplest and most effective insurance policy against such thrombosis. It does not always prevent coronary occlusion, but it is *much* the safest preventative.

Q. 18 — *Can a person with high blood pressure be treated with vitamin E?*

A.—There is much public misinformation on this point. Some hypertensive patients display a small initial rise of blood pressure when *first suddenly* given *large* doses of vitamin E. As this agent continues to be taken, any elevation of pressure may drop—although perhaps not to normal levels.

More than anything else the hypertensive fears a stroke, a blood clot or ruptured vessel in the damaged arteries of his brain. There is no safe prophylactic agent he can take to ward off this danger but vitamin E. It is his best and safest insurance policy. He needs that policy desperately and should keep his premiums paid every day as long as he lives.

(Read Chapter IX, page 40, *The Heart and Vitamin E*.)

Q. 19 — *Will vitamin E help an enlarged heart?*

A.—Enlargement of the heart is usually evidence of a weakened heart muscle. The heart compensates in quantity for a defect of quality. Hypertension and acute and chronic rheumatic heart disease are the common causes. Both of these, notably the rheumatic hearts, are much helped by taking vitamin E, but whether or not the damaged, enlarged heart shrinks depends on how much of the size increase was due to mere dilation and how much to actual increase of muscle bulk. Both may be combined, of course. Fundamentally, only dilated hearts can shrink again.

The measurement of heart size is full of fallacies. It can be done accurately only by X ray, and the technique of such X ray is open to serious question. A scanty increase in heart area represents considerable increase of volume. For example, it appears that an increase of one centimetre in transverse diameter represents a

----

doubling of the volume of the heart. It is easy to see that the heart can be greatly helped, even reduced considerably in spherical size, and yet little change may appear in the X ray picture.

Q. 20 — *What will vitamin E do for irregular heart beat?*

A.—There are many types of irregularity of the heart. Not many patients who have had auricular fibrillation for a long time will ever be restored to normal heart rhythm again, whatever drug is used. The occasional *fresh* fibrillation will be restored to normal by alpha tocopherol, howeverer. Some patients with extra systoles, which are merely dropped beats, get complete relief from these by taking alpha tocopherol.

Actually the effect of this substance is upon the heart muscle itself rather than upon the rhythm of the heart.

Q. 21 — *Is there liver impairment after heart failure?*

A.—With heart failure blood backs up into the liver, lungs, the extremities, the body cavities, and so forth. This backing up into the liver produces liver congestion and liver enlargement, liver tenderness, and presumably impairment of liver function. This last, however, is very difficult to measure, and it is questionable as to whether it produces specific clinical signs of any importance.

Q. 22 — What is meant by "coronary insufficiency"?

A.—Coronary insufficiency means inadequate circulation via the coronary arteries. This is usually due to hardening of those arteries. The arteries fill up with arteriosclerotic lesions just as a kettle limes up with sediment if one repeatedly boils hard water in it.

The net result is that a smaller current of blood flows through the bore of the coronary arteries. The muscle of the heart is relatively starved for blood and, therefore, for oxygen, and the outstanding symptom that ensues is anginal pain. This really is the heart muscle crying out for more oxygen.

Coronary insufficiency is often called coronary sclerosis, and both of them are almost synonymous with angina pectoris.

Q. 23 — *What has vitamin E to offer the swollen or waterlogged patient in heart failure?*

A.—It is often helpful. Although such a patient may be irreparably damaged, with the aid of rest and mercurial and other diuretics, digitalis, and so forth, he may survive for years. Alpha tocopherol aids the flagging heart muscle of these patients and its helpful influence on the kidneys is another benefit. Even in the worse cases of failure the injection of mercurials may be spaced farther apart when alpha tocopherol is administered, and in milder failure mercurials may sometimes be dispensed with. A word of sharp warning! Where there is a rheumatic basis for the failure, or an associated hypertension, the sudden administration of large doses of alpha tocopherol (as in certain medical experiments that have been reported) may seriously jeopardize the patient, and is most unwise. Hence the need for close supervision of such cases when you are aware of the dangers involved. Every potent medicine can be wrongly used and so make mischief. Alpha tocopherol is no exception to that rule. Wisely used it helps. We cannot stress this enough, apparently, for patients keep on trying to treat their own hearts. Especially where there are chronic rheumatic hearts or hearts in failure this can be highly dangerous. And how many heart patients really know what type of heart disease they have?

Q. 24 — *If a person has had a recent heart attack, could vitamin E be taken?*

A.—Of course, and the sooner the better. It is important to salvage as much of the incompletely damaged heart muscle as one can before this damage has persisted long enough to be irreparable, and to make the rest of the heart muscle as vigorous as possible to compensate for what damage there has been.

Q. 25 — *Is vitamin E of any value in treating a scarred heart valve with stenosis?*

A.—It is hard to say what vitamin E has to offer for a scarred heart valve with stenosis. Some scars on the palms and soles are relaxed when vitamin E is taken. No other substance has this power. The mechanism of this effect is unknown, as well as the reason why it does not happen to all scars. It is easily conceivable that some scarring of heart valves may loosen up slightly when alpha tocopherol is taken. As a matter of fact, there have been reports in the medical literature of changes in heart sounds following the administration of alpha tocopherol; this could be explained as indicating changes in the constricted valve orifices.

What is much more important is the possibility that fibrin plaques may not have the same tendency to accumulate on the heart valves during the acute phase of rheumatic infection if alpha tocopherol is taken, for it is definitely a fibrinolytic substance, the only safe one we are aware of. If no fibrin is laid down, or the fibrin is decreased in amount, the heart valves are the less likely to agglutinate and create a stenosed or narrowed orifice.

Q. 26 — *Is there any significance in the fact that the modern increase in heart trouble has kept pace with increased cigarette smoking?*

A.—Perhaps. The same studies so widely popularized and indicating so definitely the harmful influence of smoking on lung cancer demonstrated quite as clearly that heart disease rose in frequency in cigarette smokers, not in proportion to the increase in cancer, but very considerably.

We stop many heart and vascular patients smoking, because smoking a cigarette contracts the blood vessels. If the patient already has an inadequate circulation, he is foolish to jeopardize what he has left by throwing his vessels into spasm with tobacco. The smoker is about as clever as a pugilist would be who hit himself on the jaw, or a football player who turned about and carried the ball across his own goal line.

We do not say "cut down." We say: "You have smoked your last cigarette." We have even reached across to a patient's pocket, picked his cigars out of that pocket, and thrown them into the wastebasket beside us. Such a patient may be startled and slightly resentful, but he gets our meaning. And we really mean it. If he persists in smoking, it is too bad.

Q. 27 — Does vitamin E help stimulate sluggish circulation?

A.—Since vitamin E is a *vascular* vitamin effective in plasma and in the blood vessels, if "sluggish circulation" refers to some vascular insufficiency, vitamin E would be primarily helpful.

Q. 28 — *If a patient has had a thyroid operation and the heart still beats fast, would vitamin E be effective?*

A.—This fast rate is probably due to old damage to heart muscle by the once overactive thyroid. The heart must now beat oftener because it contracts less adequately each time. On account of its effect on heart muscle vitamin E should prove helpful here also. Certainly it justifies an extended trial in such patients.

Q. 29 — *We read much these days about coronary heart disease. Is this a comparatively new disease?*

A.—So it seems. Coronary thrombosis was first reported at autopsy in 1898, although angina from coronary sclerosis had been known for nearly two centuries before. Sir James McKenzie, the founder of modern cardiology, died in 1925. In his day, he saw most of the important cardiac patients in Great Britain and Europe. In his book on angina pectoris, he stated that 380 patients consulted him for angina pectoris in his whole lifetime. Contrast this figure with that of the modern cardiologist, who counts his coronary patients by the hundreds.

Q. 30 — *Is it true that electrocardiograms have the same individuality as fingerprints?*

A.—No. There is a distinctive finger-print pattern for each person, but no such wide variety of electrocardiograph tracings is possible. However, there is a characteristic pattern for many types of heart lesion, and this pattern, taken in conjunction with the patient's history, can be very informative or even diagnostic. Certain types of cardiac disease, such as heart block, can be diagnosed in no other way.

Q. 31 — *What advice is given heart patients about dieting?*

A.—Our doctors take the view that diet in terms of foods providing *nourishment* is a better therapeutic investment than diet in terms of restriction. About the only nutritional advice formerly offered to those who wished to avoid coronary heart disease was: "Never become overweight, and if you are overweight, reduce." More recently this advice has been modified, because it has been found that unless he *stays* reduced, he may do himself more harm by repeated loss of weight than by staying moderately overweight.

We have commented before on the general confusion regarding fats in the diet and especially cholesterol. Until much more is known we think it is foolish to attempt to curtail the average man's diet. However, to be on the safe side, and in order to remain at least on the edge of the current of modern medical thought, we often suggest a restriction of total fats and especially of animal fats, even the addition of 3 ounces of corn oil to the daily intake—but we are far from convinced that this has any major benefit to offer a man who is already damaged about as much as he can be by decades of an arteriosclerotic process, and is now sufficiently deteriorated to present symptoms. Moreover, any diet he is given must be maintained for the rest of his life, perhaps for twenty years more. Otherwise it is futile. What restrictive diet is he apt to follow for such a period of time, at every meal, every day (unless he is a diabetic and is compelled to do so for mere survival), especially when he reads that investigators currently differ widely among themselves as to the need for such restriction?

Q. 32 — *If one gives vitamin E, may he give any other drug with it?*

A.—Certainly, you may give almost anything else at the same time. Doctors regularly prescribe digitalis, nitroglycerine, mercurial diuretics, and so on, along with vitamin E. Just as those who use penicillin do not discard iodine or alcohol swabs or cleanliness, so one would be foolish to disregard the valuable features of traditional heart treatment and replace them at once and routinely with alpha tocopherol. Many patients must always take digitalis with alpha tocopherol; some need mercurials for years as well. But many people gradually find digitalis or mercurials no longer needed or required in smaller doses, or less often. *Iron tonics should be avoided at the same time as alpha tocopherol is being taken. If taken together the effect of the vitamin E being given seems to be destroyed.* If insulin is used simultaneously with alpha tocopherol, insulin reactions should be watched for, as the patient's need of insulin may suddenly be decreased at any time. Unsaturated fats, notably cod liver oil and animal fats, should probably be reduced or excluded from the diet when one takes alpha tocopherol. Unsaturated fats increase the need for vitamin E; saturated fats destroy it in the body.

There are two qualifications of these remarks that could be made at this point.

(a) One can take *organic iron,* such as is found in raisins, spinach, or in many other foods, or as an organic iron salt, at the same time as he takes vitamin E, and no harm is done to the tocopherol. It is *inorganic iron,* such as most iron tonics contain, that seems to destroy vitamin E by oxidation.

(b) If one gives iron because of a profound anemia, for example, he can still give it when vitamin E is being administered by separating the doses of each in the stomach. That is, one can take all his vitamin E at or before breakfast and all his inorganic iron at bedtime—or vice versa. Thus an interval of at least eight hours separates them, and the inorganic iron does not oxidize the tocopherols in the stomach.

Iron can be given by intramuscular injection at any time, of course. It is only iron in the bowel that interacts with vitamin E.

If one is giving a vitamin-mineral mixture at the same time as vitamin E, he should be sure to find out if the iron in it is the permissible organic or the improper inorganic type.

Q. 33 — *If a heart patient takes a daily dose of a form of digitalis, may vitamin E be taken at the same time?*

A.—Yes, by all means; many do. But, remember, it is easier now to get a digitalis overdose. The two drugs work in similar fashion on the enzyme systems of the failing heart muscle. Therefore a dose of digitalis one has given for years may soon become an overdose when one gives vitamin E; an overdose of digitalis can produce confusing and harmful effects. It can nauseate the patient, alter his electrocardiogram, and so on. This is why all patients taking digitalis, and especially digitalis plus vitamin E, need regular medical supervision by a careful doctor who is aware of this new problem.

Q. 34 — *I have been giving an anticoagulant, dicumarol, since a coronary attack. Do I dare to give vitamin E at the same time?*

A.—Yes, if you decide to do so. But if you give vitamin E, you need no longer give the dicumarol, which is dangerous in any case and of very dubious merit. Vitamin E, can replace it promptly, completely and safely if used in proper quantity.

However, patients can make these changes only under medical supervision and must not assume the responsibility of doing so on their own. We warn patients very stringently against such rashness.

Q. 35 — *After starting vitamin E therapy, must one continue indefinitely thereafter? Would there be bad after-effects if one stopped giving it?*

A.—If one starts to eat bread he always needs bread. If a man starts to eat steak and potatoes the body continues to need them. Vitamin E is just another food. If one begins to take it, he wonders how he ever got along without it. If he stops it, the effect soon wears off, as is true of bread and meat. The influence of any food is usually transient.

If the patient stops it, in a matter of a few days, he returns to much the same condition as before.

The patient is under no compulsion to take vitamin E at any time, just as one really is not compelled to eat anything. But people who stop eating regret it, and that is true of vitamin E also.

Vitamin E is treatment, not cure—like insulin, for example. The day the diabetic stops his insulin he becomes the same old diabetic he was before he took insulin. This is true of cardiovascular patients taking vitamin E. In a few days or weeks after it has been stopped, the patient once again is vulnerable and exposed to the steady ravages of his disease.

He should keep taking his vitamin E. There is no insurance policy so simple, safe, cheap and easy. Don't let his premiums lapse.

Vitamin E is not habit-forming.

Q. 36 — *What can one do for low blood pressure?*

A.—Nothing. It is probably an asset. Some of the greatest athletes have had it and thrived. In any case, almost certainly nothing valuable and permanent can be done to elevate that low reading, unless it be a facet of a constitutional, debilitating disease. Then the disease itself needs treatment, not just the "low blood pressure."

Q. 37 — *Does one's blood pressure change with age?*

A.—Probably a gradual, steady rise occurs as a person ages. This is one of the points now being re-evaluated by the medical profession.

Q. 38 — *Does a heart murmur always mean a diseased heart?*

A.—Not by any means, although it often points to old rheumatic heart infection. "Functional" murmurs are occasionally found. These change with exertion or bodily posture. Some infants have such murmurs that soon disappear. But any murmur should be investigated for it may be highly significant.

Q. 39 — *A person gets breathless on the stairs or when hurrying for a bus. Is this due to heart trouble?*

A.—It may be. Many other causes of breathlessness, such as asthma or other lung diseases, even anemia, can produce the same disability. The doctor must decide if early heart failure is impending—or if this breathlessness is quite unrelated to heart disease.

Q. 40 — *A person is considerably overweight. Does that affect his heart?*

A.—It gives his heart more work to do. It has been estimated that for every twenty pounds of extra weight one carries the heart must push blood through twelve extra miles of blood vessels. This is an added burden on any heart that is already flagging. Why put such a strain on a heart? Reduce his weight and have him *stay slim*.

*_ _Circulatory Diseases of the Legs_

....Circulatory Diseases of the Legs

Q. 41 — *Is vitamin E used to treat varicose veins?*

A.—We originally refused to treat such patients, thinking it was absurd to believe that vitamin E had anything to offer them. But so many patients with such leg conditions, whom we treated for other cardiovascular diseases, told us how much their varices improved that we finally decided it was worthy of trial, and now we have become thoroughly convinced of its value.

How could it possibly be helpful?

To answer this one must briefly describe the probable cause of most varicose veins. This description is over-simplified, perhaps, but then there is considerable disagreement among authorities as to the detailed mechanisms involved. Fundamentally there are two sets of leg veins, the superficial set one sees at a glance, and the deep set running through the depths of the great muscles of the leg. The latter set is designed to carry about 85 to 90 percent of the return flow from the feet, the former only 10 to 15 percent. If the deep set becomes obstructed by old phlebitis, for instance, a new load falls on the superficial set which was never designed to handle such an excess. In the effort to do so the superficial veins distend, dilate, twist and become "varicose," as we say. Then their valves become useless or nearly so, because the valve cusps are pulled apart as the veins enlarge, "communicating veins" from the deep set pour blood into them steadily, and the full weight of a tall column of venous blood bears on the thinned-out vein walls of the feet and lower legs. At this point we say that the patient has varicose veins in full bloom.

Along comes an ambitious surgeon. He sees the legs and suggests that they are unsightly and need an operation on the veins. Once on a time he would have suggested injection, but the result of injections proved to be so poor that these are now rarely done. Then came the era of ligation (tying off the veins in several places in the thigh and leg). There were so many recurrences after this operation that now it, too, is rarely done. At the moment the fad—and these seem to be fads—is for "stripping." The results of this operation are often poor, too, for after about a year or a year and a half varicose veins recur, as they should and must. For these are the veins in that superficial set that the patient desperately needs, inadequate as they are, and new varicose veins *must* reform to permit something like an adequate return flow from the feet and legs.

We never suggest surgery for varicose veins, therefore— except for women who are ashamed of their unsightly big varices—but advise the use of alpha tocopherol instead. It acts on such legs by an altogether different principle.

It mobilizes collateral or detour circulation about the obstructed veins in the deep parts of the leg. These, therefore, take some of the burden off the existing superficial, varicosed set of veins. The appearance of the latter may or may not be improved—but there is less swelling, less pain and ache in the lower legs, and the natural tendency of the veins to worsen should be halted. Sometimes, too, there is an obvious improvement in the appearance of these legs, but we never promise it. That is an "extra" when it occurs.

Certainly everyone with varicose veins should try vitamin E before he considers operation—and should also remember how poor the results of operation usually are. We see people who have had three and four series of such operations, and end exactly where they began.

Q. 42 — *What does vitamin E have to offer in phlebitis of the leg?*

A.—It is the best and safest agent one can use. It not only melts away the existing clot and helps the inflammatory process to subside, but it hinders extension of that process and almost never permits a part of the clot to break loose and strike some other part of the body, such as the lungs or brain (an accident called embolism).

There are many anti-clotting agents one can now give when there is a clot in a blood vessel, but none are safe. They all tend to overdo their job and produce hemorrhages. These bleedings can be serious or even fatal, and such complications of the use of anticoagulants are now everyday accidents throughout the country.

We feel that vitamin E is very effective in preventing thrombosis within the vascular system, and acts more simply, more cheaply, and much more safely than the rival anticoagulants. The safety factor is very marked, indeed, as is the simplicity of this vitamin E treatment. It requires no stay in hospital, no repetition of blood clotting tests, can be self-administered by mouth

under a physician's occasional direction—*and
never produces hemorrhage*. Perhaps the best
argument for it, however, is the power that medical writers have generally ascribed to it to min-
imize embolism. One of the most serious dangers
in having a clot develop in any vessel is the risk
that a piece of it will break loose and plug some
vital and distant organ, for example the brain or
lung.

We let our peripheral thrombosis cases do
ordinary work and be normally active throughout
treatment, just because we are so sure that no
embolism will develop, and because inactivity so
often tends to induce further thrombosis as the
blood current slows down during bed rest.

If a thrombosis case does not respond rapidly
(within three to five days) to vitamin E therapy,
it merely suggests to us that the dose we gave has
been inadequate and we promptly increase it.
One gives the dose needed to do the job.

Vitamin E should be continued for at least two
weeks after the clinical cure of the patient, and
for some the dosage continued almost indefinitely thereafter. The reason is that for years
thrombosis tends to recur, perhaps from a blow
on a chair leg or the kick of a grandchild, or even
after a cold or other simple infection. Vitamin E
is preventive as well as curative, and is a

valuable insurance policy against recurrences. The more numerous the recurrent attacks the greater the final sum of vascular damage to the leg and the more apt that patient is to become a "chronic" case with constant peripheral pain, swelling, ulceration and general disability.

Q. 43 — Should a man with Buerger's disease take vitamin E?

A.—He certainly should, if he stops tobacco, for nothing else has much to offer him.

Buerger's Disease affects men nearly exclusively, and consists of a gradual impairment of circulation in the terminal twigs of the arteries of the extremities, particularly the legs. This is ascribed to a clotting process there. It often shows itself first in young men (below 50 years of age) who develop recurrent leg thrombosis, or cramps in the legs upon exertion (claudication). Tobacco makes it worse, and most of these men are smokers. Women almost never develop this condition. Some recent writers have regarded it as a form of arteriosclerosis. Certainly if it is, it is an unusual type, with certain peculiarities all its own.

The gradual and very painful process of obliteration of circulation in the tips of the toes and fingers may go on to a gangrene which eventually involves all the extremities and leads to multiple amputations. The disease usually attacks the brain and heart eventually, and many of these patients mention early loss of memory and suffer particularly intractable coronary accidents.

Vitamin E in proper dosage gives good and prompt relief of the leg symptoms, including the cramps which develop on walking, the thrombosis or gangrene, but does little for the loss of memory and such. Certainly every Buerger's patient should use vitamin E, because alternative treatments are very discouraging, and here is a simple, cheap and effective alternative. It is also *absolutely essential to stop tobacco*. No one who continues to smoke is apt to get relief.

Q. 44 — *A patient has had a leg ulcer for 15 years. It heals and breaks down time after time. Now it has become very painful, and is surrounded by an area of reddened, very itchy skin. Can vitamin E help him?*

A.—Yes, vitamin E is able to give him at least as much help as any other treatment.

Most such ulcers are caused by defective circulation in the leg, perhaps on the basis of hardened arteries, old chronic phlebitis producing an obstruction of venous outflow and hence a chronic congestion of the lower leg. Often the two conditions are combined. Then a blow or other injury produces an ulcerated area, which becomes infected in a part of the body exposed to soiling and difficult to care for. The result is a painful, chronic, discharging, foul ulcer. It may persist and give trouble for twenty to thirty years, eventually becoming almost crippling. The size of the ulcer seems to have little bearing on the pain it produces.

This ulcer must be cleaned up and kept clean, perhaps with hot whirlpool baths, perhaps with the additional use of antibiotics or other antiseptic agents. Then as much circulation as possible must be restored by means of vitamin E, and a certain amount of postural drainage is indicated. It may be wise to elevate the leg higher than the head several times a day (lying on the floor with the leg on a chair) in order to cut down the chronic congestion. Arterial damage may not permit this, however, and may render the distress in the leg tolerable only when the leg hangs down out of bed or from a chair.

In any case vitamin E should be applied

locally in spray or ointment form and taken orally in large doses. Many people cannot tolerate the ointment very well on such tender, devitalized skin and can use it only in much diluted form, vaseline being the diluent. If the ointment can be tolerated, however, the local application of vitamin E is of great help.

Not only must such an ulcer be healed but *it must be kept healed*. This means it should always be protected with a pad of gauze or by some other means, and a continuing dose of vitamin E should be given in order to maintain the improved circulation it originally induced as well as one can. The recurrences develop in people who ignore this precaution.

Q. 45 — *A patient has a huge leg, due not to venous obstruction but to obstruction of lymphatic channels. Can vitamin E help her?*

A.—Not much, if at all. Perhaps you have been misled, however, for it is very hard to make such a pronouncement with surety. Many a so-called lymphoedema, producing what we call elephantiasis of the leg, has elements of venous thrombosis in it as well as of lymphatic obstruction. The two types of channels run side by side, and one is often involved when the other is (although this may be masked by swelling), and one really never knows what the total situation is until he tries vitamin E for its effect on any *venous* obstruction present.

A trial for two or three months of what vitamin E has to offer is always indicated, therefore, since no other practical and simple measure can be suggested by anyone. Certainly surgery seems to be disappointing.

Q. 46 — *An old man has pain in his legs at night. It awakens him about four o'clock or earlier, and he gets relief only by getting up and walking about the room. This is not a muscle cramp or knot, but a severe, steady ache. What can I give for relief?*

A.—Vitamin E is your best hope. This complaint is probably due to arteriosclerosis or Buerger's disease, the same difficulty in supplying his legs with blood which used to give him cramps in the calves of his legs or thighs when he walked, but which he ignored then or for which he has received no help. Now it has progressed to give him pain at rest, because at rest the bloodflow is slowed and his feet and legs complain of being cheated of blood and the oxygen that that blood distributes.

He can restore arterial (inflow) circulation by walking, by holding his legs down over the side of the bed, or by vitamin E—but his condition could be so advanced that perhaps nothing but amputation can give him relief.

He must never smoke again, assuming that he does, since tobacco closes down his arteries, and closed arteries are the crux of his problem.

Q. 47 — *A man has just had a "stroke." Does vitamin E have any value in the treatment of such cases?*

A.—Yes, a great deal of value. A "stroke" is often just another blood clot, this time in a certain set of vessels near the base of the brain. What has been said about alpha tocopherol helping clots in other blood vessels applies equally here. If given to a case of apoplexy early, there may be quick recovery and a good deal of it. Less recovery ensues the longer treatment is delayed, as could be anticipated, but even some late palsies are helped very obviously.

Best of all, its prophylactic values are important. For if one has had one stroke, he merely awaits the second, and so forth. Vitamin E is a simple, cheap, safe insurance policy against that repeated apoplexy.

Q. 48 — *It seems silly to use vitamin E in cases of gangrene. Do you do so?*

A.—This is one of the most valuable uses of alpha tocopherol. For gangrenous areas originally die, and dead or gangrenous areas spread, because of a lack of arterial blood inflow and consequent oxygen starvation of the tissues nearby. Only measures designed to increase these factors can alter gangrene for the better. Alpha tocopherol is the best of all such agents. We have repeatedly published observations on the benefits derived from vitamin E treatment in such patients, and other workers have abundantly confirmed our findings.

Certainly any gangrene caught in time, especially in a diabetic, is apt to be controlled or even saved from amputation by the administration of vitamin E. We wish it were tried routinely. It should be.

Unfortunately, it is so often used when it is too

late, when there has already been so much damage to the arteries supplying an extremity and such prolonged blood starvation of the part that no salvage is possible. This should not be called a failure of vitamin E but merely an impossible problem in chronic tissue starvation.

Vitamin E cannot do impossible things, though it is often called upon to try.

If an extremity has to be amputated for gangrene, it is increasingly important to salvage what is left. As *the original arteriosclerotic process still goes on* to attack the other toes or the other leg this patient *now more than ever* should be urged to take vitamin E. He must try to protect what he has left. His problem is not solved. Indeed, it has now become more urgent than ever, for he has more need of his remaining members. We find it difficult to convince people of this obvious point.

Q. 49 — *A patient occasionally has numb, tingling fingers. Is that due to arteriosclerosis or defective circulation?*

A.—Almost certainly not. This numbness is usually an early manifestation of neuritis and responds rapidly to the administration of large doses of vitamin B₁ (thiamine chloride), given either orally or by intramuscular injection or both.

Q. 50 — *An old patient has been advised to have an arterial graft for his arteriosclerotic leg. Should he?*

A.—Be very cautious about such an operation and treat it as a last resort. At the moment many of these grafts immediately clot, which can precipitate an emergency in the circulation of the treated limb. Strangely enough, too, many grafts gradually become arteriosclerotic in their turn. The results are apt to be much poorer a year after operation than immediately after it, therefore, and this defect of the graft becomes even more obvious as more time elapses. One should be pessimistic about surgical relief, therefore, particularly when vitamin E provides such a good and safe alternative measure.

Why not wait for that graft till vitamin E has been tried?

Q. 51 — *What about vitamin E for Raynaud's disease?*

A.—Raynaud's disease, the paroxysmal spasm of the digital arteries, produces pallor or cyanosis of fingers or toes. It can be precipitated by uncontrolled emotional upset and cold, and is most prevalent in young women and in men who use tobacco.

Vitamin E is very useful, indeed, the most helpful treatment. But we always suggest a warm climate and avoidance of needless stress as well. Large doses of vitamin E are needed, however— and needed permanently.

Q. 52 — *A child of six has albumin and red blood cells in the urine, and has been diagnosed as having acute nephritis. Does vitamin E help such cases?*

A.—Very little is known about the treatment of acute nephritis and usually doctors have little to suggest. Fortunately 85 percent to 90 percent of these cases seem to cure themselves spontaneously, in time. Vitamin E has been used by us in the treatment of these patients, sometimes with spectacular success. The medical literature contains thirty-two papers besides our own, papers coming from Italy, France, Spain, England, India, Germany, Portugal, suggesting that this is good treatment.

Certainly vitamin E deserves an intensive trial in such patients.

Q. 53 — *A little girl has been badly burned. The wounds are nearly healed but skin grafting has been suggested.*

A.—It is *most unfortunate* that vitamin E, both locally and orally, was not used as soon as the child was burned. Burns constitute one of the best indications for the use of alpha tocopherol, for it heals such wounds rapidly and the wounds heal without scarring and scar *contraction*. No other agent has this power. The absence of scarring and scar contraction obviates the need for any or much grafting, and grafting is always unsightly.

Grafting may be indicated, but remember that the grafts will "take" better and with less scar disfigurement if vitamin E is given by mouth and applied locally at the same time.

If a burn is at a later stage and the wounds have healed to produce raised scars (keloids) that are very itchy or "burn," vitamin E applied locally usually gives wonderful relief quickly.

The main thing to remember, now and in the future, is that vitamin E is the best treatment for burns at any stage and should *always* be used.

_Uses in Obstetrics, Gynecology, Urology and Pediatrics

......Uses in Obstetrics, Gynecology, Urology and Pediatrics

Q. 54 — *A girl has pain at menstruation. What has vitamin E to offer her, if anything?*

A.—It has long been known that taking vitamin E for several days before a period often relieves menstrual pain. Large doses are rarely needed.

Q. 55 — *Can vitamin E help regulate menses?*

A.—Depending on the medical reasons for irregular menstruation, vitamin E might well have a positive effect. It is a customary finding that pain and cramps during a period can be reduced. Like so many other marginal problems, vitamin E should be tried for period irregularity. That is the best way to find out its effect.

Q. 56 — *I have heard that vitamin E is merely a "sterility vitamin." Is that so?*

A.—Originally, from 1922 on, vitamin E was called the "sterility vitamin" because it prevented rats from aborting. It does so many other much different things, however, that this property now seems less important. We feel that its obstetrical values have constituted a considerable handicap to its use in many other unrelated conditions just because they were unrelated. This is a mental hurdle in the medical mind that has been hard to overcome. This often misguided description of vitamin E has held back serious research on the vitamin by twenty years.

Q. 57 — *Does vitamin E help male impotence and male infertility?*

A.—Rarely one hears of some relatively impotent man whom vitamin E seems to help. We suspect this effect is largely mental. Certainly no one need fear to take it because of sexual over-stimulation. That *does not occur*.

Vitamin E has been used for male infertility, because it seems to improve the *quality* of

----

sperms. It is very doubtful if it improves female infertility, however. We often administer it to a husband before conception occurs, in the hope of rendering any subsequent pregnancy more normal, and especially for guaranteeing a normally formed baby. We believe it is always wise to do so, particularly if any previous child has been malformed— with a cleft palate, spina bifida, or other such defect.

Q. 58 — *Is vitamin E helpful in the menopause?*

A.—There are more medical papers advising the use of vitamin E in the menopause than for any other medical condition. In relatively small doses it often decreases the severity of hot flushes and the headaches occasionally encountered at this epoch. It is not as effective for hot flushes as estrogens—but never makes the patient bleed and therefore wonder if she has cancer of the uterus. It can safely be used in patients with a cancer background— unlike the rival estrogens.

Q. 59 — *Does vitamin E prevent miscarriage?*

A.—It has long been used for that purpose and

seems to be at least as effective, if used promptly and in adequate dosage, as any other known substance.

Moreover, it is as effective in preventing premature delivery as in miscarriage. It has saved many babies from being born too soon, even after the membranes have ruptured too early. Since prematures so often die or are hard to raise and very trying, vitamin E should always be administered from the beginning to the very end of pregnancy, and especially to women who have terminated pregnancy too soon in earlier conceptions.

Doses used for the complications of pregnancy are usually much less than are demanded by cardiovascular conditions.

Q. 60 — *Does vitamin E help prevent birth defects?*

A.—It is likely that giving vitamin E to the sire before conception improves the subsequent chances of the birth of a normal infant.

Q. 61 — *A woman has chronic rheumatic heart disease, and now is two month's pregnant. Can she carry the child; will she need Caesarean, or will she have a normal birth and normal baby?*

A.—This is a large and complicated question, but it can be answered rather briefly. Much depends upon whether the disease of this heart is severe or mild. But most people can carry on with one or a few such pregnancies *under special care,* can deliver normally rather than by Caesarean, and can have a good baby. Usually labor is considerably easier and faster in cardiac mothers.

It is certainly true that such a patient needs the best kind of obstetrical care, both before and during delivery. She may feel unable to undertake too many pregnancies, which makes the children she does have unusually precious, and this, in turn, makes even clearer the need for the *best medical care* before, during and after pregnancy.

Q. 62 — *A woman has been told she is Rh negative. Does that interfere with taking vitamin E?*

A.—Her Rh negative status is entirely irrelevant to vitamin E. Her Rh factor seems to matter only in respect to transfusion or to the life, health or death of her children—and then only if her husband is Rh positive.

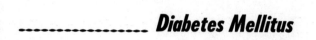 *Diabetes Mellitus*

Q. 63 — What are the symptoms of untreated diabetes mellitus?

A.—There is characteristic thirst and increased output of urine. There may be localized or generalized itching of the skin or genitals, loss of weight, loss of libido. Sometimes the disease is first recognized when gangrene of the toes appears, or when a woman develops a vaginitis which is intensely itchy and is due to thrush. Often a plague of boils heralds the disease, or infections that the individual finds hard to throw off. An elevated urine sugar and blood sugar confirm the diagnosis, of course.

Q. 64 — Does vitamin E help diabetes?

A.—It should always be taken, we feel. It is now

quite widely believed that diabetes is a two-phase disease, one aspect being characterized by a high blood sugar, the other by vascular degeneration. All that one does by controlling the former is to lay bare the latter. It is for this reason that vitamin E is particularly useful. For not only is it occasionally able to lower the elevated blood sugar somewhat, and therefore decrease the requirement of insulin, but it looks after the unrecognized and insidious vascular complications of the disease which all fear. Nothing else is so well able to give the diabetic insurance against the vascular ravages of his disease, the retinal hemorrhages, coronary disease, kidney complications, claudications and gangrenes that so inevitably come on in twenty or twenty-five years of diabetes.

Diabetics on insulin taking vitamin E may suddenly find they require less insulin and may have an insulin reaction on the dose they have long been taking. Therefore, we warn diabetic patients first going on vitamin E to keep honey handy in order to ward off any such difficulties.

Q. 65 — Can vitamin E be used for diabetic cataracts?

A.—It is usually ineffective here, unfortunately.

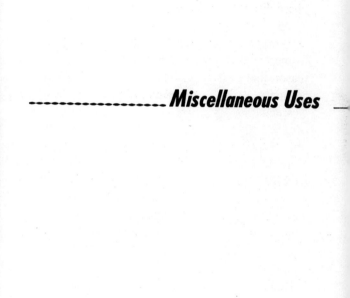

-------------------- *Miscellaneous Uses* ___

----------------*Miscellaneous Uses*

Q. 66 — *Can vitamin E be toxic?*

A.—There are several therapeutic applications which require skilled administration of vitamin E. In healthy people, there are no known toxic effects or side effects. This is one of the distinctive characteristics of vitamin E.

Q. 67 — *Is it possible to have an allergic reaction to vitamin E supplements?*

A.—Yes, some people have sensitivities to oil-base material. These include persons with malabsorption. There is nothing in our experience to suggest that vitamin E itself can cause allergic reactions. Such reactions are caused by the "vehicle" used to carry the vitamin E material into the stomach. This vehicle is usually vegetable oil, and those allergic to it may experience minor discomfort in the form of a mild rash on the torso or transient upset stomach. Severe reactions are unheard of. Since some marketers of vitamin E use mineral oil as the vehicle, this would, of course, compound the reaction problem.

Q. 68 — *Can the body manufacture vitamin E?*

A.—No, only plants can synthesize vitamin E. This is why nutritional intake of vitamin E depends on the intake of vegetables and grain, not animal tissue.

Q. 69 — *Why is vitamin E associated with anti-aging?*

A.—One of the recent developments in the understanding of vitamin E is that it is a regulator, controlling the rate at which blood platelets clot, controlling the release of histamine in wound sites and also the rate at which tissue deteriorates. Since aging is synonomous to tissue deterioration, this is how vitamin E effects aging.

Q. 70 — *Does vitamin E have any value in eye diseases?*

A.—We are scarcely competent to answer that question, as we have very little first-hand experience of what it does in these conditions.

However, there are many papers in the medical literature suggesting that it is helpful in some examples of a variety of eye complaints, for example, the rare cataract, the occasional degeneration of the macula, and notably, hemorrhagic retinas. We ourselves have seen and known of such cases, and believe alpha tocopherol should always be given to such patients, notably those with hemorrhages in the retina, not only to help resolve what blood has already clotted there, but also to improve the walls of the retinal capillaries to such an extent that they will not rupture again.

Actually we doubt that the values of this agent in ocular disease have as yet been adequately explored.

Q. 71 — *Has vitamin E any value in psoriasis and eczema?*

A.—Rarely, if ever, is psoriasis helped by the administration of alpha tocopherol.

"Varicose ecxemas" are often helped, espe-

cially by the local application of vitamin E ointment in patients whose skin can tolerate it. What
it can do for other "eczemas" is unpredictable,
but a cautious trial in stubborn cases may occasionally be indicated.

But the principal value of vitamin E in skin
conditions is in collagenosis, the leathery skin
around ulcerated or chronically phlebitic ankles.
It rarely relieves this, but it prevents its continued progression and its encroachment on adjacent areas (for this condition usually goes on to
girdle both ankles gradually. Then it is crippling.) No really helpful answer to this situation
has ever been suggested before.

**Q. 72 — *What does vitamin E have to
offer cases of "polio," or muscular
diseases in general, for example,
muscular dystrophy, progressive
muscular atrophy, and so on?***

A.—Here, again, not too much is known. Rats
whose mothers are deprived of vitamin E soon
display a characteristic muscular dystrophy after
birth. This dystrophy responds to vitamin E
treatment. Other animals, such as rabbits and
guinea pigs, also show experimental muscular
dystrophy. But the human is different, for some

reason as yet unknown, and his muscle dystrophy does not respond to alpha tocopherol, at least in the usual dosage which experimenters have tried.

Some polio cases are helped by vitamin E, even in the chronic stages, both in respect to muscle power and as regards the cramps and aches in their muscles. Acute cases certainly justify a trial of vitamin E, but very little is known of what it has to offer them.

Progressive muscular atrophy does not appear to respond to vitamin E.

Q. 73 — *Does vitamin E help arthritis?*

A.—Only in the small joints of the hands. When vitamin E ointment is rubbed into such hands this arthritis is often much helped. For larger joints it appears to be ineffective as a primary treatment. As a secondary (or accompanying) treatment, vitamin E most regularly reduces pain in the joints.

Q. 74 — *What value has vitamin E in leukemia?*

A.—None, unfortunately.

Q. 75 — What value has vitamin E in lupus erythematosis?

A.—We have seen several cases. Some are not helped and some are much improved.

Q. 76 — Is vitamin E helpful in myositis?

A.—The vitamin E ointment rubbed into the sore muscle and tissues, and then the local application of heat, are often very helpful measures.

Q. 77 — Does vitamin E help Dupuytren's contracture?

A.—Dupuytren's contracture is a contracture of the fingers caused by the shortening of the deep muscles of the palm. In chronic cases, scar forms and the hand freezes in a claw.

Vitamin E is at least as helpful as surgery. Often considerable relaxation of such old palmar scarring is seen, even after years of disability. But often it seems to do nothing at all for particular patients.

Q. 78 — What about vitamin E in thyroid function?

A.—We are still uncertain of the answer here. When an overactive thyroid is present, we use it very watchfully. In underactive thyroid states there is no contraindication, of course.

Q. 79 — Is vitamin E helpful in acne vulgaris?

A.—This is the disease of 100 cures. Occasionally vitamin E ointment is worthy of a brief trial. It rarely helps.

Q. 80 — What value has vitamin E in Peyronie's disease?

A.—A great many papers in the medical literature advise its use in this condition (plaque formation along the lateral and dorsal aspects of the penis, resulting in curvature, painful intercourse and discomfort.) We have seen very few cases, but most have been appreciably helped by vitamin E.

Q. 81 — What role does vitamin E play against cancer?

A.—Not much is understood about the use of

vitamin E in the treatment of cancer. It is, however, safe to say that there is no direct effect
because there is no direct relation between
vitamin E's role as a vascular agent and the onset
of cancer. Vitamins A and C have shown their
strength in cancer treatment, and since vitamin E
is synergistic with both these vitamins, there is
an indirect connection of vitamin E to cancer
treatment. This is one aspect where there is little
biochemical or clinical data. But for patients
about to be exposed to irradiation, topical and
oral administration of E is suggested.

Q. 82 — *Is vitamin E recommended before surgery?*

A.—As a vascular vitamin, vitamin E intake is
absolutely indicated for all potential patients.

Q. 83 — *In treating burns and lacerations, is it more beneficial to the skin to take vitamin E orally or to put ointment directly on the skin?*

A.—For most household burns and cuts, vitamin
E ointment is best. Some people who don't have
vitamin E ointment at the time, break open a
capsule of the acetate. It is better advice to use

the ointment for topical applications. The use of oral vitamin E with the application of the ointment is the procedure for more serious burns and lacerations. The ointment is specifically designed for use on the skin. Most ointments have 30 mg per gram, and are made of acetate vitamin E in a vaseline-like base.

Q. 84 — *Does vitamin E work with vitamin C in the prevention of colds?*

A.—Yes, vitamin C and vitamin E are complementary.

Q. 85 — *Does vitamin E have any relation to mental capacity? To emotional disposition?*

A.—Vitamin E is a vascular vitamin. If there is some limitation of mental capacity due to poor blood supply, then vitamin E would be directly helpful. It has been used successfully in the treatment of cerebro-vascular impairment. Usually, mental capacity is limited more by neural insufficiency and in that case the B vitamins would be best applied.

The disposition of an individual is even more

complex, and determination of the effect of vitamin E is almost impossible. Supplementation of any substance cannot ensure relaxation or the joy of life. The only direct connection I know of is that a person who is healthy (and vitamin E does encourage good health) is likely to feel well-disposed toward life. This is one of the goals of preventive medicine.

Q. 86 — *What is the difference between natural and synthetic vitamin E?*

A.—Natural vitamin E can be derived from a number of vegetable oils by a distillation process. Natural Vitamin E is chemically called d-alpha tocopherol as it only occurs as the d- molecular configuration.

Synthetic vitamin E is produced from isophytol, a petroleum or turpentine product. It is chemically called dl-alpha tocopherol as it contains both the d- and l- molecular configurations (isomers).

Natural-source vitamin E has a higher level of biological activity than synthetic vitamin E. The l-form of alpha tocopherol was found to have only 21 percent of the biological activity of the natural d-alpha tocopherol.

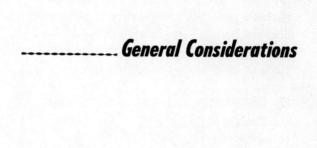

General Considerations

--------- General Considerations

Q. 87 — What is an isomer?

A.—An isomer is a compound which has the same molecular formula as another compound. They have the same number and same kinds of atoms, but the atoms are attached to one another in different locations.

d-alpha tocopherol and 1-alpha tocopherol are examples of isomers as their molecular formula is identical, but their spatial arrangement of atoms is different.

Q. 88 — What are the acetate and succinate forms of vitamin E?

A.—Acetate and succinate are organic substances naturally found in our bodies. In preparing vitamin E, they are frequently combined with vitamin E to provide natural resistance to oxidation and spoilage. Acetate is derived from acetic acid, which is common vinegar. Succinate is derived from succinic acid, which is commercially derived from acetic acid. Both acetic and succinic acids lose their mildly acidic properties upon combining with vitamin E.

Q. 89 — *What does esterfied vitamin E look like? What does it do?*

A.—The molecular structure of a substance can be made more stable by a chemical procedure. In the case of vitamin E this can be noted on the label of the material when a d alpha tocopherol becomes esterfied to d alpha tocopheryl. This leaves the vitamin E more resistant to loss of potency when exposed to storage, sunlight and heating.

Q. 90 — *Can we be sure of getting enough vitamin E in our daily diet without taking it separately?*

A.—"Vitamin E" is there, but in small quantities only. The principle available sources are whole wheat bread (one that really is not just white flour discolored with molasses) and margarine prepared from vegetable oils (not containing animal fats). The amount of *alpha tocopherol* (the most active fraction) in even this sort of supplementary diet would be small (less than 7 milligrams per day) and of little or no value for therapy. It might be prophylactic over the course of many years.

I suppose if one ate a great deal of natural wheat he might obtain as much ''vitamin E'' as he would require. But he would have to eat a very large bulk indeed, would have stomach room for very little else, and we're afraid the diet would prove monotonous. It seems to be much more reasonable to make up for the deficiency of years by taking a small volume of a highly concentrated oil (alpha tocopherol in capsule form) which contains much the same elements. Supplementation remains the least expensive manner to meet even the nutritive RDA (15 mg for adults in the case of vitamin E), let alone seeking a prophylactic (a dosage to reduce ancestral susceptability to vascular reduce ancestral susceptability to vascular disease) or therapeutic intake.

The average American or Canadian ingests about 10 to 12 mg of *alpha tocopherol* per day. He absorbs much less, after cooking—perhaps 6-8 mg daily. But his daily requirement has been estimated at 20 to 170 mg per day. It is easy to see that a deficiency could develop in a man so cheated of his requirement over a period of forty to sixty years. Eating a little vegetable margarine would be slow to compensate for those starved years.

Q. 91 — *Does vitamin E work in concert with other nutrients?*

A.—With vitamins A and C, vitamin E supports the assimilation of most other nutrients. Healthy tissue absorbs nutrients better than deficient tissue. However, the relationship of vitamin E to other food factors is not as strong as it is with vitamins A and C.

Q. 92 — *What vitamins or foods destroy vitamin E or inhibit its effectiveness in the body?*

A.—It is not so much what food as what kind of food. Research has shown that there are only 1.19 mg alpha tocopherol in prepared frozen dinners. Foods fried in animal fats as is common in fast-food restaurants create a much greater need in the body for vitamin E; foods fried in vegetable oil do not necessarily raise the need, but the vitamin E present in the oil is destroyed in the cooking. Mineral oil destroys vitamin E.

Q. 93 — *What foods contain vitamin E?*

A.—Common vegetables and grains of all kinds contain proportionately large amounts of vitamin E. Muskmelon, peaches, spinach, salmon, almonds, butter, raw sunflower seeds, safflower oil, sesame seeds, wheatgerm, sprouts, filberts, eggs, asparagus are especially good sources.

Q. 94 — *Is vitamin E always destroyed in cooking?*

A.—Some vitamin E can resist breakdown up to 115 degrees F. Generally, only 15 percent of vitamin E remains after typical American cooking. It is not as resistant to good freezing.

Q. 95 — *What about storing vitamin E? Can it go bad?*

A.—Vitamin E is oxidized in the presence of sunlight. This is why an esterfied form of vitamin E (see question 88) is best for storage.

Q. 96 — *Should vitamin E be included in the diet of pets?*

A.—Animals benefit greatly from some intake of vitamin E. Animal breeders, animal research farms and those who raise animals for competition (most notably racehorses) commonly use vitamin E. It has a direct effect on coats of fur-bearing animals. Mink farms customarily use vitamin E supplementation in feed rations. Dosage for animals can be computed on the basis of 30 mg per kilogram of weight.

Q. 97 — *Do you feel that mixed tocopherols are required along with alpha tocopherol?*

A.—There are seven known tocopherols, but the most active by far is alpha. Beta has about two-thirds of its activity; delta and gamma are relatively inert. The three new tocopherols that were discovered in 1955 are as yet largely unknown quantities in pharmacy.

All natural tocopherols are mixtures of the seven; indeed, it is impossible to find a natural tocopherol which is pure alpha. On the other hand, since alpha is much the most important constituent, the efficacy of such a mixture is assayed and should be stated in terms of its alpha activity. It is really the alpha fraction that matters, so far as cardiovascular disease is concerned at least.

Q. 98 — *Does vitamin E provide energy?*

A.—In some people, there is a marked energizing influence on physical exertion. For others, there is no discernable effect. We tell patients to be watchful for the effect, and to save the energy—not use it to stay up later to tend to household chores.

Q. 99 — *Why do athletes take vitamin E?*

A.—One of the roles of vitamin E in the blood plasma is to enable the blood to carry more oxygen per unit volume. Since vitamin E also regulates oxidation (use of oxygen) throughout the body as well, these two effects are what athletes and race horses look for.

Q. 100 — *Should infants and growing children take vitamin E?*

A.—Definitely.

Q. 101 — *What amounts of vitamin E per day would you recommend for an apparently healthy individual?*

A.—The crux of this question is in the word "apparently." A person who is apparently well may be in reality far from well. One of the best examples of this we have seen was the partner of a great professional skater who came to us several years ago with very marked damage to his chronic rheumatic heart. When he maintained himself in good condition for his professional skating career his heart compensated well and he had no obvious signs of heart failure. But when he got out of condition he began to relapse. "Apparently" healthy people, therefore, may not mean healthy people.

Perhaps everyone's dose differs, and should be personally adjusted, as he ages, and with regard to his type of activity.

The dose of vitamin E one requires depends intimately on his blood pressure and any evidence he may have (perhaps is unaware of) of chronic rheumatic heart disease.

In addition, the apparently healthy person must first answer what he seeks from a supplemental intake of vitamin E or any other food

factor. Dose varies from nutritive use to prophylactic use to therapeutic use.

Q. 102 — *What are the factors that determine individual need for vitamin E?*

A.—Biological individuality is customarily dis-
regarded to some degree in our American com-
munity. Unless there is some obvious side-
effect, formulas have been designed to be applied
to almost any situation. The skill of physicians
working with vitamin E and in the whole field of
"preventive medicine" is that a large variety of
possible reactions to or deficiencies in vitamin E
are looked for. People develop different needs
for vitamin E if there is a positive vascular history, if diet is insufficient, if there is an intolerance
or malabsorption of oils or if living under smog.
Smokers destroy at least 400 units of vitamin E
per day. There are any number of variables
which would determine an individual's need for
vitamin E.

Q. 103 — *What is your opinion about the objection that too many claims are made as to the powers of vitamin E?*

A.—If one objects that too much is claimed for it, we could remind him of ACTH and cortisone which, although much newer, have already been used for *hundreds* of varying disease conditions. Or we could remind him of the tranquilizers, of Indian snake-root, and a host of new additions to the pharmacopeia. In fact, it sometimes seems that we moderns have reverted to the old days of "shot-gun therapy" when one prescription was aimed at almost everything. This objection to the multiple powers of alpha tocopherol, therefore, scarcely holds. This argument is presented only by those who do not know enough about vitamin E to understand that it is a *vascular* vitamin. Its effects are simply limited to those disorders stemming from complications in the blood or blood vessel. We have never suggested it was good in inflammatory or neural or viral disabilities, for instance. This agent should be valuable wherever circulation or oxygenation can be improved in the body, and everyone knows that he has blood vessels from the roots of his hair to his toe nails, and that improved circulation or better oxygen supply are as apt to help the pregnant uterus as the damaged heart, the damaged brain or damaged skin.

Q. 104 — *What is vitamin E oil?*

A.—Vitamin E oil is a pharmaceutical preparation having some percentage of vitamin E acetate in a "vehicle" of vegetable oil.

Q. 105 — *What is your opinion of wheat germ oil?*

A.—We wish it were off the market. It is so dilute and so readily deteriorates that it can play little if any part in good treatment. It lulls the patient into false security as he often takes it in good faith, thinking he is taking vitamin E in proper form and quantity. If you were to follow the milling of wheat germ, you would see that the slight heat of the rollers is sufficient to render tocopherol (an alcohol) diffuse. The only vitamin E in wheat germ is to be found in the walls of the room where it is milled.

Q. 106 — Why does the Shute Institute recommend such high dosages of vitamin E when the MDR is only 30 mg for adults?

A.—It is important to realize that the MDR of any vitamin or mineral is that amount necessary to sustain life. The MDR has nothing to suggest in the nutritional supply of a vitamin, for the prophylactic supply or the therapeutic applications in deficiency states. Thus, 30 mg of vitamin E will support life in tissue, but offers no additional effect. It is worth noting that the typical North American diet supplies less than half the MDR for vitamin E. This is one reason we suggest that people should take 800 units of vitamin E per day so that there will be sufficient supply in the body to diffuse and prevent deficiency.

Q. 107 — I can prescribe much cheaper brands of vitamin E in the United States than you recommend. Are you aware of this?

A.—Yes, we have long known it;—but we still

recommend only ethical products which we have seen tested.

It is possible, by means of tricky labelling, to sell 100 units of "vitamin E" when the capsule really contains 46 to 136 international units of alpha tocopherol acetate, the form of vitamin E active in cardiovascular disease. "Vitamin E" is merely medical slang. What we are concerned with in our treatment is *alpha* tocopherol.

At least it is obvious that there may be three times as much alpha tocopherol in one capsule as another, depending on the tricks of labelling. This permits a price spread of 300 percent between market products showing the same label strength, i.e., "400 units."

Now we must suggest only the products of ethical companies, that is, pharmaceutical firms that contact physicians to tell them about such medicinal agents as vitamin E, and also maintain laboratories where they can produce new products and standardize them. These ethical companies spend huge sums in producing literature for doctors and in keeping a staff of representatives on the road and in doctors' offices. Only thus can doctors be told of vitamin E and learn to use it: *We look forward to the day when more doctors know of it, use it, and can treat all their clien-*

tele. That day will come only when ethical companies have convinced them about vitamin E.

But it costs money, as has been said, to organize and maintain such a firm. The ethical companies charge more for their vitamin E products than do little companies which merely have a room over a garage or food store in which they can store bottles and from which they can ship mail orders. These companies do nothing to promote the cause of vitamin E. They merely ride on the backs of the pharmaceutical houses that do, and on our backs. As long as marketers dominate the field, patients will continue to have trouble being treated by vitamin E at all or only after making long trips to see such doctors as have used it for years and understand it.

Which shall it be—a bargain price for the patient and no doctor to help him—or a reliable product which costs slightly more and every doctor ready to use it? Each must decide when he buys his next bottle of vitamin E. *This is not our problem only;* why should we alone struggle with it with the help of a few ethical companies? It is really the problem of government agencies which have no real care for vitamin E and less regulatory curiosity.

Q. 108 — *Why do so many physicians look askance at vitamin E? Has the use of vitamin E in heart disease been thoroughly documented?*

A.—Physicians have their own reasons for resisting the obvious uses of vitamin E. Vitamin E has always been known as good medicine but bad for business. It is safe to say that customary medical learning never has included study of the vitamins and never will unless there is pressure from the public for its doctors to become more familiar with them. This is in fact what has begun to happen. We give credit for this to ''people power.''

There has never been an instance in previous scientific history where thorough documentation (by this I assume you mean crossover double-blind research) has really proven anything to anyone who was initially critical or changed the attitudes of a single critic. Even the critics know how easy it is to develop statistical data to support any point of view. To wait for a mass of medical documentation to sway the collective mind of the physician is like holding a candle into the wind.

What is needed is that vitamin E be tried once

fairly by each and every physician who wants to know if vitamin E will effect a given patient. To try it for a vascular complaint is to prove whether it works or not. Therein is the answer.

Although the tide has swung, it has always been a characteristic of the vitamin E controversy that the real question up for grabs was *not* whether the material worked or whether it didn't. It should be remembered that while the idea of vitamin E is not new to some of us, it is an idea barely thirty years old. Vitamin E has just come of age. Although I doubt I shall live so long, present generations will see the acceptance of vitamin E. Its time has come.